Rachida Lamiri
Nahla kechiche
Ibtihal Jamal

Local recurrence of nephroblastoma

Rachida Lamiri
Nahla kechiche
Ibtihal Jamal

Local recurrence of nephroblastoma

Predictors of local recurrence in nephroblastoma

ScienciaScripts

Imprint

Any brand names and product names mentioned in this book are subject to trademark, brand or patent protection and are trademarks or registered trademarks of their respective holders. The use of brand names, product names, common names, trade names, product descriptions etc. even without a particular marking in this work is in no way to be construed to mean that such names may be regarded as unrestricted in respect of trademark and brand protection legislation and could thus be used by anyone.

Cover image: www.ingimage.com

This book is a translation from the original published under ISBN 978-620-6-72510-7.

Publisher:
Sciencia Scripts
is a trademark of
Dodo Books Indian Ocean Ltd. and OmniScriptum S.R.L publishing group

120 High Road, East Finchley, London, N2 9ED, United Kingdom
Str. Armeneasca 28/1, office 1, Chisinau MD-2012, Republic of Moldova, Europe
Managing Directors: Ieva Konstantinova, Victoria Ursu
info@omniscriptum.com

Printed at: see last page
ISBN: 978-620-8-35504-3

INTRODUCTION

Nephroblastoma or Wilms' tumour is a malignant tumour that develops at the expense of embryonic renal tissue [1, 2, 3, 4, 5].Wilms' tumour reproduces nephrogenesis, and all 3 components of the differentiating metanephros can be observed: undifferentiated blastomeres, epithelial structures and connective tissues or various mesodermal derivatives (mesenchymal or stromal) [6, 7, 8, 9]. It is the most common malignant renal tumour in children aged between 1 and 5 years (more than 90% of renal tumours in children) [1, 2, 6].It may be discovered following palpation of an abdominal mass (95% of cases), or in the presence of other signs such as abdominal pain, haematuria, fever or changes in general condition [5, 8, 9, 10].The diagnosis of nephroblastoma is based essentially on radiological investigations (ultrasound and abdominal CT) [2, 4, 6, 11].An ultrasound- or scan-guided biopsy is sometimes used for diagnostic purposes in doubtful cases [12].Nephroblastoma is the tumour that has benefited most from therapeutic advances, based essentially on surgery, chemotherapy and even radiotherapy [2, 13, 14]. The stage of extension is defined on the basis of the radiological assessment of extension, the operative report and the anatomopathological examination of the surgical specimen [6, 7, 10]. Local recurrence (in 20% of cases) or metastases (pulmonary or hepatic) are possible [4, 8, 12]. They should be detected by quarterly surveillance including a clinical examination, chest X-ray and abdominal ultrasound [14].

Local recurrence poses the problem of its aetiology, which is multi-factorial, represented essentially by: under-classification of the tumour, inadequate pre- or post-operative chemotherapy, surgical error (tumour rupture, failure to resect peritoneal-diaphragmatic or parietal residues), and unfavourable histology.

The aim of this study was to investigate local recurrence of nephroblastoma. Local recurrence is defined as recurrence of the mass in the original tumour bed, retroperitoneal or within the abdominal cavity [15]. Thus, in the light of 14 cases of local recurrence of nephroblastoma collected in the paediatric surgery department of the Fattouma Bourguiba University Hospital in Monastir, between 1995 and 2012, we propose to study:

-Epidemiological, clinical and therapeutic features of local recurrence of nephroblastoma.

- Factors predictive of local recurrence.

- The prognosis for these 14 recurrences.

PATIENTS AND METHODS

This is a retrospective study of 14 cases of local recurrence of nephroblastoma collected in the paediatric surgery department of the Fattouma Bourguiba University Hospital between 1er January 1995 and 31 December 2012.

The study involved all cases presenting to the department with a clinical, radiological and histological diagnosis of nephroblastoma, and having recurred locally after surgery, as well as cases presenting at the stage of local recurrence.

Epidemiological, clinical, radiological and anatomopathological data, as well as the various treatment methods, results and evolutionary aspects were collected from the clinical files using an analysis form. This essentially included: the patient's medical and surgical history, the circumstances in which the pathology was discovered, the results of the clinical examination and additional biological and radiological tests, the treatment methods: surgery and pre- and post-operative chemotherapy. These analysis sheets also specify patient follow-up, the circumstances in which local recurrence was discovered, the medical and surgical treatment adopted, the progress made under treatment and the follow-up period. In our study, we adopted the classification of the different stages of extension according to SIOP 2001 (appendix).Statistical analysis was carried out using the Statview version 5 package. The descriptive study was expressed as percentages and represented graphically in the form of pie charts. Using the decision tree, we have found that the most suitable tests for this study are The "Fisher Exact Probability" for the study of the correlation between the qualitative and quantitative variables, and the "Linear Correlation Coefficient" for the study of the correlation between the quantitative variables, with a statistical significance threshold set at P

< 0,05.

I- EPIDEMIOLOGY

From 1 January 1995 to 31 December 2012, 115 cases of nephroblastoma were treated in the paediatric surgery department of the Fattouma Bourguiba University Hospital. Among these patients, 14 had presented with a local recurrence of nephroblastoma after curative surgery, representing an annual incidence of recurrence equal to 0.82 cases per year and a frequency of 12%.

I-1-AGE

The age of our patients ranged from 3 days to 9 years, with an average of 4.5 years (Figure 1).

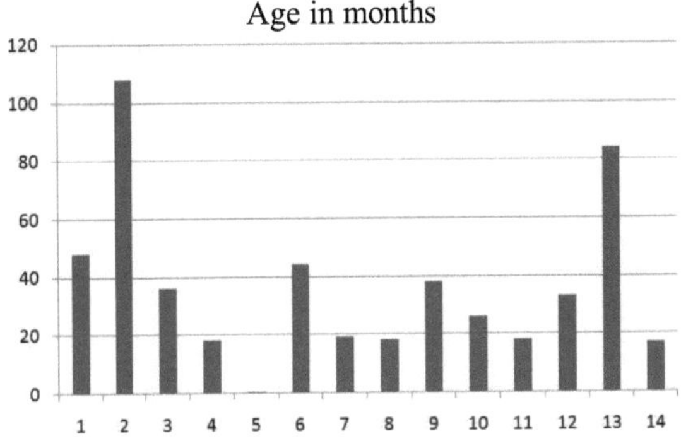

Number of cases

Figure 1: Age distribution of patients.

The age group less than or equal to 3 years (36 months) was the most affected, accounting for 57% of cases.

I-2-SEX

Ten patients were female (71%) and 4 male (29%), with a sex ratio of 0.4.

I-3-FAMILY HISTORY

Only one patient had a maternal uncle who died of a renal tumour at the age of 5. In the 13 other cases, none of the patients had a family history of carcinology.

II- INITIAL TUMOUR

II-1-CLINICS

II-1-1-CIRCUMSTANCES IN WHICH NEPHROBLASTOMA IS DISCOVERED

The abdominal mass was the main reason for discovery. It was found in 13 cases (92.8%) (Table I).

Table I: Circumstances in which nephroblastoma is discovered.

	Frequency	Percentage (%)
Abdominal mass	12	92,8
Abdominal pain	4	28,6
Haematuria	1	7
Weight loss	2	14,3
Fever	2	14,3

The sum of percentages greater than 100% is explained by the possibility of two or three signs being associated in the same patient.

II-1-2- CLINICAL EXAMINATION

Abdominal examination revealed an abdominal mass in the left hypochondrium in 54% of cases, in the right hypochondrium in 23.5% of cases, and finally in the left flank, right flank and right iliac fossa in 7.5% of cases each. Palpation of the mass was sensitive in 2 cases (14.3%) and painless in 12 cases (85.7%). It revealed a poorly limited mass in 5 cases (38.5%) and a well limited mass in 8 cases (61.5%). The mass was fixed in all cases. The size of the mass on palpation varied between 5 and 15 cm, with an average of 10 cm. All patients had a normal rectal examination (no nodules or palpation of the lower pole of the mass) and were in good general condition.

II-2- ADDITIONAL DIAGNOSTIC TESTS FOR NEPHROBLASTOMA

II-2-1-ABDOMEN WITHOUT PREPARATION

PSA was carried out in 8 patients, and there were no abnormalities in any of them, in particular no bone lysis or calcification.

II-2-2-ABDOMINAL ULTRASOUND AND ABDOMINO-PELVIC COMPUTED TOMOGRAPHY

Ten patients underwent ultrasound and abdominal-pelvic CT. Abdominal and pelvic CT scans were performed alone in 4 patients These radiological investigations showed a tissue tumour, abdominal in thirteen cases (93%) and abdomino-pelvic in one case (7%). In all patients, the mass was retroperitoneal and more precisely of renal origin, left in 9 cases (64%) and right in 5 cases (36%) (Figures 2 and 3).

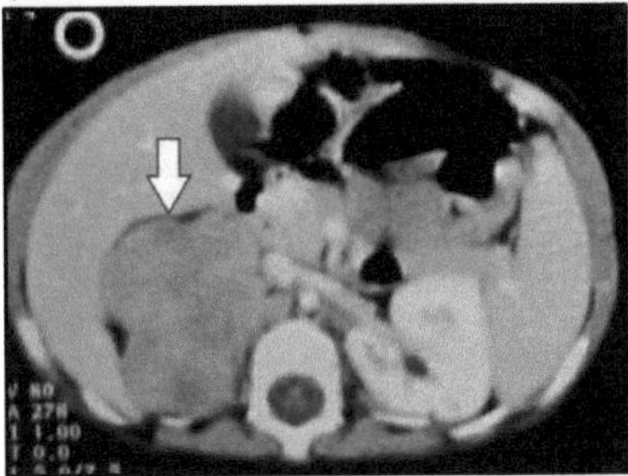

Figure 2: Abdominal CT (APC): Tissue mass over the right kidney.

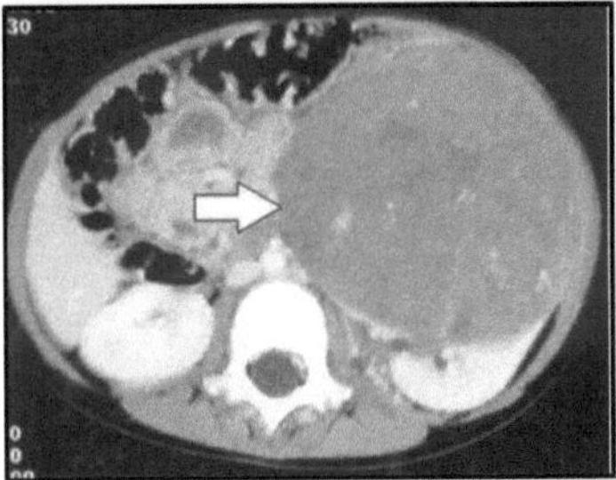

Figure 3: Abdominal CT scan (APC): Retroperitoneal tissue mass adjacent to the left kidney with spur sign.

The initial size of the tumour ranged from 60 mm to 150 mm long axis, with a mean of 105 mm. Calcifications in the tumour mass were observed in 3 patients (29%). These were either scattered macroscopic calcifications or central punctiform calcifications.Only one patient presented with multiple bilateral medullary-cortical lesions that were iso-dense and not contrast-enhanced, with a mass 60 mm in diameter on the left kidney, in favour of a nephroblastoma of the left kidney on a bilateral renal nephroblastomatous lesion.Based on the ultrasound and scans, the diagnosis of nephroblastoma was accepted in all cases. Only one patient underwent a scan-guided biopsy for diagnostic purposes because he had not responded to 4 weeks of pre-operative chemotherapy, with even an increase in the size of the initial tumour.

II-2-3-BIOLOGY

Urinary VMA metabolite assays were carried out in 4 patients whose results fell within the normal range.Biological renal function was normal in all patients.

II-3- ASSESSMENT OF EXTENSION

The extension work-up included a full clinical examination and additional radiological examinations.

II-3-1-CLINICAL EXAMINATION

Clinical examination revealed no HMG, SMG or ascites in any of the cases. The lymph nodes were free in all cases, except in one patient who presented with a firm right inguinal adenopathy 1 cm in diameter.

II-3-2- CHEST X-RAY

Chest X-rays were performed in eleven patients (79%), and showed no detectable abnormalities.In the remaining 3 patients, a thoracoabdominal CT scan was performed immediately.

II-3-3-ABDOMINAL ULTRASOUND AND THORACIC-ABDOMINAL-PELVIC CT SCAN

These radiological examinations made it possible to diagnose metastases in 3 patients, i.e. 21% of cases.
Of these 3 patients :

- 2 had pulmonary metastases (the first had 8 diffuse sub-centimetre nodules in both lung fields (Figure 4), while the second had multiple diffuse macro-nodules in both lung fields)
- one had a liver metastasis (2 liver nodules measuring 1.5 and 2.5 cm) (Figure5).

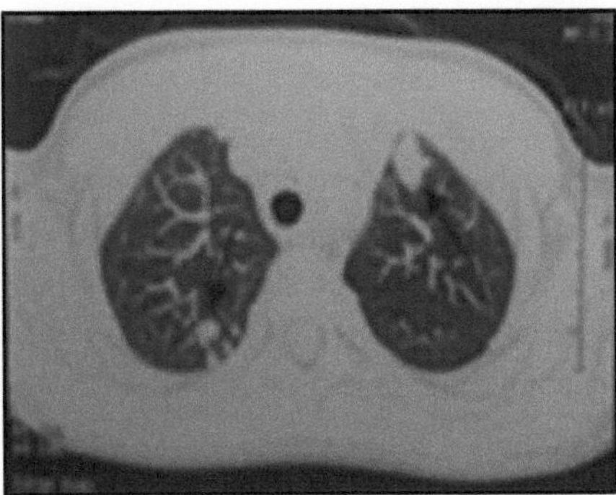

Figure 4: Thoracic CT scan: pulmonary metastases in the form of diffuse sub-centimetre nodules in the 2 lung fields.

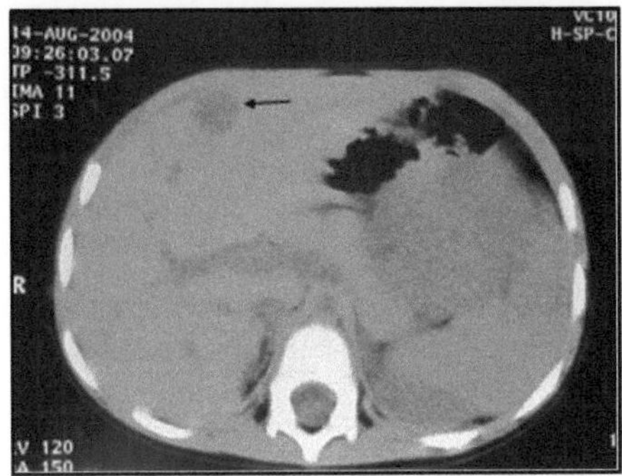

Figure 5: Abdominal CT scan: segment IV liver nodule, 15 mm, subcapsular.

II-3-4 - ABDOMINAL DOPPLER ULTRASOUND

Doppler ultrasound was performed in eight patients, and in all cases showed no venous thrombosis (RV and IVC).

II-4- TREATMENT

II- 4-1-PREOPERATIVE CHEMOTHERAPY

Thirteen of our patients underwent pre-operative chemotherapy (93%). One patient underwent immediate surgery due to strong suspicion of a mesoblastic nephroma (Bollande tumour).

a- Anti-cancer drugs

Three types of drug combinations were used in our patients: 1ère combination:

Oncovin + Actinomycin

2ème combination: Adriamycin + Vincristine + Actinomycin 3ème combination: Oncovin + Actinomycin + Epirubicin.

Of the 13 patients who received pre-operative chemotherapy, 5 had received the 1ère combination (39%), 3 had received the 2ème combination (23%), 2 had received the 3ème combination (15%) and 3 patients for whom the medical treatment was not specified (23%).

b- Duration of chemotherapy

The duration of chemotherapy varied between 4 and 8 weeks, with an average of 5 weeks.

c- Response to chemotherapy

- **The tumour response :**

In 11 out of 13 patients, partial regression of the tumour was observed, with the percentage of regression varying between 50% and 80%, with an average of 65%. (Table II)

Table II: Tumour response to preoperative chemotherapy.

	Frequency	Percentage(%)
Partial regression	11	84
Stable	1	8
Worsening	1	8

- **The response to metastases :**

Distant metastases had disappeared in 2 patients (one lung metastasis and one liver metastasis). One patient retained a right pulmonary nodule.

II- 4-2- CURATIVE SURGERY

a- Surgical removal

All our patients underwent open surgery. The approach was a wide transverse incision above the right or left umbilicus, depending on the location of the tumour (Figure 6).

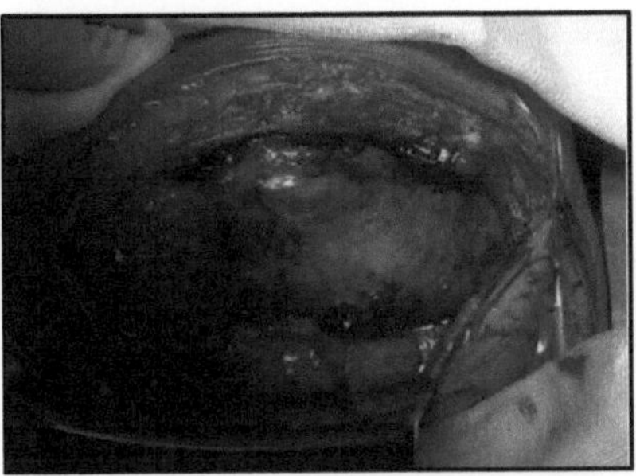

Figure 6: A large transverse incision above the left umbilicus.

Surgical excision was complete, i.e. enlarged ureteronephrectomy in 13 patients (Figure 7) and partial left excision in one patient who presented with a left nephroblastoma on a bilateral renal nephroblastomatous lesion.

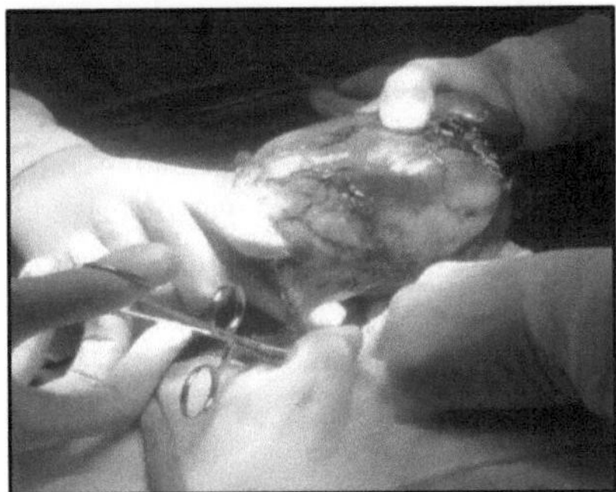

Figure 7: Final stage of a left enlarged uretero-nephrectomy involving ligation of the left ureter closest to the bladder.

Adenopathy sampling was carried out in all cases except in 2 patients, for whom no adenopathy was found. A Redon drain was placed in the renal pelvis in 3 patients (21%).

b- Difficulty in surgically removing the tumour

Surgical excision in 7 of our patients was considered difficult (50%), due to multiple adhesions with the wall, diaphragm and various neighbouring organs.
On the other hand, surgical removal of the remaining 7 patients was considered easy. It was noted that in no case did the renal capsule break intraoperatively.

c- Post-operative care

All our patients had a simple post-operative course.

II-4-3-ANATOMOPATHOLOGICAL EXAMINATION

a- Stage of tumour extension

The majority of cases (43%) were classified as stage I. (Table III)

Table III: Stage of tumour extension.

	Frequency	Percentage
Stage I Stage II Stage III Stage IV	6 3 2 3	43% 21,5% 14% 21,5%

b- Histological types of tumour

Nine patients had a mixed histology, and 5 patients had a predominance of the blastematous component. Capsule overshoot was observed in 8 out of 14 patients.

c- Anaplasia

Only three patients had anaplasia on pathological examination.

d- Venous thrombosis

No neoplastic venous thrombosis was observed.

e- Tumour weight

The weight of the tumour was not specified in 11 cases. In the 3 remaining cases, the average weight of the tumour was 1670 grams.

II-4-4- POST-OPERATIVE TREATMENT

a- Chemotherapy

Thirteen of our patients had received postoperative chemotherapy (93%).

One patient did not receive preoperative chemotherapy because of the strong initial suspicion of mesoblastic nephroma, and postoperative clinical and radiological monitoring was decided (because the tumour was classified as stage I, N0, M0).

⇨ Anti-cancer drugs :

Three types of combination therapy were used in our patients: $1^{\text{ère}}$ combination: Oncovin + Actinomycin.

$2^{\text{ème}}$ combination: Adriamycin + Vincristine + Actinomycin. $3^{\text{ème}}$ combination: Oncovin + Actinomycin + Epirubicin.

Of the 13 patients who received postoperative chemotherapy, 4 had received the $1^{\text{ère}}$ combination, 7 had received the $2^{\text{ème}}$ combination and 2 patients had received the $3^{\text{ème}}$ combination of chemotherapy.

⇨ The number of treatments :

The number of courses of treatment was not specified in 7 cases. It varied between 4 and 8 courses of treatment, with an average of 6 courses in the 7 other cases.

⇨ Duration of chemotherapy :

The duration of chemotherapy varied between 4 and 28 weeks, with an average of 16 weeks.

⇨ Response to chemotherapy :

- **The response in the renal pelvis :**

Twelve out of 13 cases had a favourable outcome (92%). One had a local worsening (recurrence of the mass on the follow-up abdominal scan performed 3 months after surgery).

- **The response to metastases :**

Of the 14 cases studied, only 3 had metastases, of which only one patient had a pulmonary metastasis (a single nodule in the right lung parenchyma) that persisted after preoperative chemotherapy, and which persisted even after postoperative chemotherapy.

b- Radiotherapy

Carried out in a single patient with stage III anaplastic disease. The course of the disease was favourable, as demonstrated by the follow-up abdomino-pelvic CT scan (one free left renal compartment).

c- Surgical treatment of metastases

Surgical excision was performed on the patient whose lung metastasis persisted after pre- and postoperative chemotherapy. A right posterolateral thoracotomy was used to perform a metastectomy. Anatomopathological examination of the surgical specimen confirmed its metastatic nature.

III- TUMOUR RECURRENCE

III-1- CIRCUMSTANCES OF DISCOVERY

Radiological surveillance (ultrasound and/or abdomino-pelvic CT scan) was the reason for the discovery of the recurrence in 12 patients. In the remaining 2 patients, an abdominal mass was discovered on clinical examination (Figure 8).

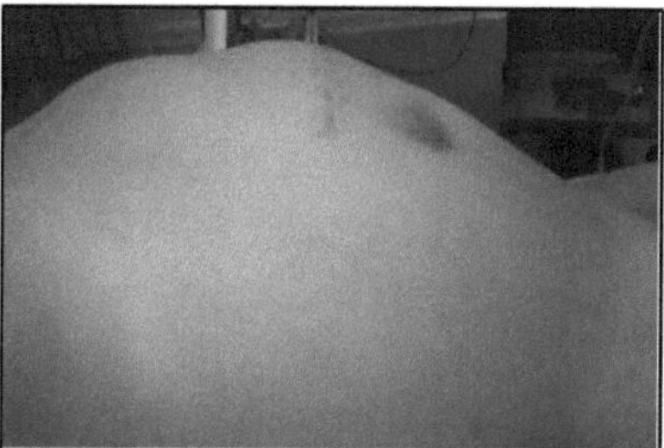

Figure 8: Showing abdominal distension due to the recurrent mass, with scar from a transverse left supraumbilical incision.

III-2- PERIOD BETWEEN THE DETERMINATION OF THE RECURRENCE AND NEPHRECTOMY

The time to local recurrence of nephroblastoma after curative surgery ranged from 3 months to 48 months, with an average of 25.5 months.

III-3-LOCATION OF RECURRENT TUMOURS

Local recurrence of the tumour was isolated in 9 cases, associated with lung metastasis in 4 cases, and associated with liver metastasis in one case. The local recurrence was either retroperitoneal on the right or left, or intraperitoneal, or of abdominal origin with a point of origin that was difficult to specify. Retroperitoneal recurrence was the most common site, accounting for 79% of cases (Figure 9).

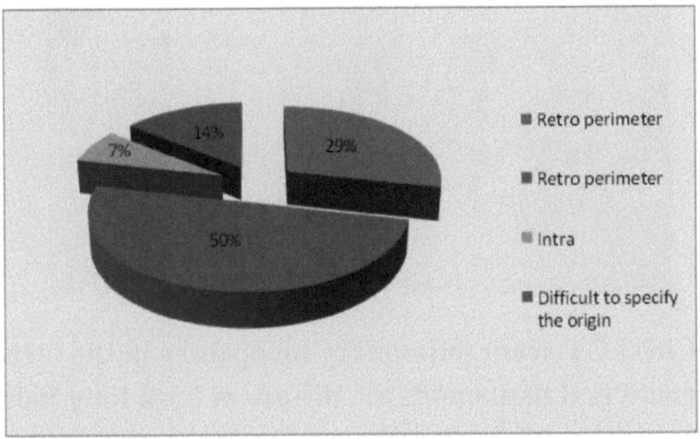

Figure 9: Distribution of patients according to location of tumour recurrence.

The size of the mass varied between 40 mm and 170 mm, with an average of 105 mm. It was well limited in 6 cases and poorly limited in 8 cases.

III-4-EXTENSION REVIEW

III-4.1. ABDOMINOPELVIC ULTRASOUND AND THORACO-ABDOMINOPELVIC CT SCAN

These radiological examinations led to the diagnosis of metastasis in 5 out of 14 patients.

Among these 5 patients, one had a hepatic metastasis (nodule of the hepatic dome measuring 2 cm in diameter), and 4 had pulmonary metastases, who presented respectively with the following lesions:

• 2 sub-centimetre nodular lesions of the right lung parenchyma.

• Subpleural micronodules in the right middle lobe.

• 5 diffuse nodular lesions in both lung fields (one on the left and 4 on the right).

• Multiple bilateral intra-parenchymal tissue nodules, peripheral and para-mediastinal. (Figure 10)

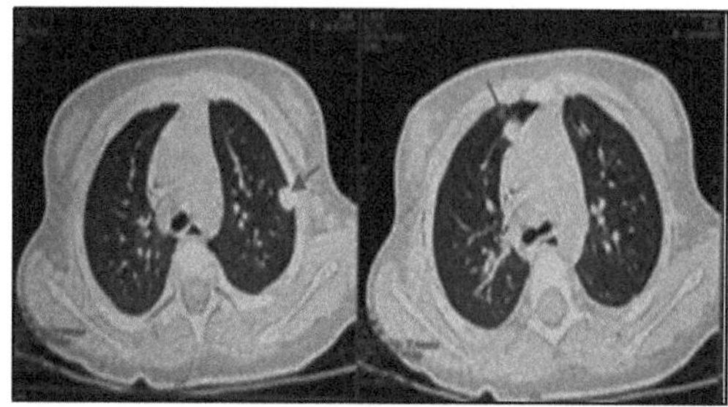

Figure 10: Chest CT scan: pulmonary metastases in the form of intra-parenchymal tissue nodules, diffuse in both lung fields.

III-4.2 ABDOMINAL DOPPLER ULTRASOUND

Doppler ultrasound was performed in 7 patients, confirming the absence of venous thrombosis.

III-5- TREATMENT OF TUMOUR RECURRENCE

III-5-1- PRE-OPERATIVE CHEMOTHERAPY

Thirteen out of 14 patients received pre-operative chemotherapy (93%), and only one patient did not.

This patient showed no response, even partial, to preoperative chemotherapy, so curative surgery was indicated straight away, as the tumour was localised and resectable.

⇨ Response to chemotherapy :

- **The tumour response :**

Of the 13 patients who underwent pre-operative chemotherapy, partial regression was observed in 10 patients, a stable appearance in 2 patients and local worsening in one patient.

- **The response to metastases :**

Local tumour recurrence was accompanied by metastases in different sites in 5 patients. There was complete disappearance of metastases in all cases except in one patient in whom there was tumour progression with bilateral pulmonary lesions.

III-5-2- SURGERY FOR TUMOUR RECURRENCE

Surgical removal of local tumour recurrence was performed in 10 patients (78%). It was macroscopically complete in all cases.

Three patients were deemed inoperable (the tumour was very large, very adherent in 2 cases and associated with peritoneal carcinosis in one case).

Only one patient did not require recurrence surgery, given the almost complete regression of the tumour size (from 90 mm to 10 mm) under pre-operative chemotherapy.

III-5-3- POST-OPERATIVE CHEMOTHERAPY

All our patients had received postoperative chemotherapy.

⇨ Response to chemotherapy :

- **The tumour response :**

Progression was favourable in 10 patients and unfavourable in 4 (tumour progression at the initial site or metastasis).

- **The response to metastases :**

Of the 14 cases studied, 5 had local recurrence associated with metastases in different sites. Complete disappearance of metastases after preoperative chemotherapy was observed in all patients except one, who showed tumour progression with bilateral pulmonary lesions.

III-5-4- RADIOTHERAPY

None of the patients had received post-operative radiotherapy.

III-5-5- SURGICAL TREATMENT OF METASTASES

One patient underwent surgical removal of a pulmonary metastasis by right posterolateral thoracotomy. Exploration revealed a metastatic nodule measuring 2.5 cm in diameter in the middle lobe margin, and a nodule 1 cm in diameter in the anterior segment of the upper lobe. The 1 cm nodule was resected using the Wedge technique with a 2 mm safety margin. For the second nodule, located in the middle lobe ridge, a metastectomy following the periphery of the nodule was performed. Post-operative management was straightforward.

III-6- ANATOMO PATHOLOGICAL EXAMINATION (Table IV)

Ten of the 14 patients retained the same histological type (mixed or predominantly blastematous). However, 4 of the 14 patients had a change in histological type (from mixed to predominantly blastematous in all 4 cases). The mean time to recurrence for these patients was 8.5 months.Tumours with no initial unfavourable histological signs retained the same characteristics in the recurrent mass.

Table IV: Histological type of initial and recurrent tumour.

Observation no.	Histological type of tumour initial	Histological type of tumour recurrent
1	Mixed without anaplasia	Mixed without anaplasia
2	Blastematous with anaplasia	Blastematous with anaplasia
3	Mixed without anaplasia	Blastematous without anaplasia
4	Mixed without anaplasia	Mixed without anaplasia
5	Blastematous without anaplasia	Blastematous without anaplasia
6	Mixed without anaplasia	Blastematous without anaplasia
7	Blastematous with anaplasia	Blastematous with anaplasia
8	Mixed without anaplasia	Blastematous without anaplasia
9	Blastematous with anaplasia	Blastematous with anaplasia
10	Blastematous without anaplasia	Blastematous without anaplasia
11	Mixed without anaplasia	Mixed without anaplasia
12	Mixed without anaplasia	Blastematous without anaplasia
13	Mixed without anaplasia	Mixed without anaplasia
14	Mixed without anaplasia	Mixed without anaplasia

IV-EVOLUTION

Of the 14 cases studied, 10 had a favourable outcome with complete regression of local recurrence or metastases. Follow-up ranged from 3 to 92 months, with a mean of 47.5 months.On the other hand, the remaining 4 patients had an unfavourable outcome: either an inoperable tumour (initial tumour site or metastatic), or resistance to chemotherapy treatment, or both. Of these 4 patients, 2 died after an average of 21.5 months from diagnosis of the disease, and 2 were lost to follow-up after an average of 7.5 months. The prognosis for local recurrence was good in 71.5% of patients (30% of whom had lung or liver metastases) and poor in 28.5% (the extension work-up was unremarkable in the latter).

V- FACTORS PREDICTIVE OF RECIDIVISM

In our series, various factors predictive of recurrence were studied. These are essentially clinical, radiological, therapeutic and anatomopathological factors.

V-1- CLINICAL FACTORS: (Table V)

V-1-1- AGE

Our patients ranged in age from 3 days to 9 years, with an average of 4.5 years. The majority of patients were 3 years old or younger.We found that the earliest recurrence at 3 months was in the oldest child in our series (aged 9).It was also noted that the average time to recurrence was shorter in patients aged over 3 years (average time 14 months), and longer in patients aged under 3 years (average time 25.5 months). The analytical study showed a significant correlation between time to local recurrence and age (P=0.0037).

V-1-2- SEX

In our series, ten patients were female (71%) and 4 male (29%). The mean time to recurrence was shorter for male patients (mean time 14 months) and longer for female patients (mean time 25.5 months). The analytical study did not show a significant correlation between time to local recurrence and patient gender (P=0.338).

Table V: Time to recurrence and clinical factors.

Observation no.	Recidivism delay (months)	Age (months)	Gender
1	5	48	F
2	3	108	F
3	8	36	F
4	4	18	F
5	7	0,34	F
6	5	44	M
7	3	19	M
8	11	18	F
9	4	38	F
10	12	26	M
11	8	18	F
12	12	33	F
13	25	84	M
14	48	17	F

V-2- RADIOLOGICAL FACTORS: (Table VI)

V-2-1- SIZE OF THE INITIAL TUMOUR

The initial size of the primary tumour varied between 60 and 150 mm long axis, with a mean of 105 mm. It was noted that patients with an initial size greater than 110 mm had an average time to recurrence that was 7.5 months shorter, and that patients with an initial size of 110 mm or less had an average time to recurrence that was 25.5 months longer. The analytical study showed a significant correlation between time to local recurrence and initial tumour size (P=0.0047).

V-2-2- DISTANT METASTASES

Three of the 14 patients had distant metastases (2 lung and one liver). The mean time to recurrence was shorter in the case of metastases, at 8.5 months, compared with the relatively longer mean time of 25.5 months in the absence of metastases. The analytical study showed no significant correlation between time to local recurrence and metastases (P=0.9814).

Table VI: Time to recurrence and radiological factors.

Observation no.	Recidivism delay (months)	Size of initial tumour (mm)	Distant metastases
1	5	140	Pulmonary
2	3	150	0
3	8	160	Pulmonary
4	4	110	0
5	7	100	0
6	5	125	0
7	3	105	0
8	11	110	0
9	4	110	0
10	12	125	0
11	8	125	0
12	12	90	Hepatic
13	25	110	0
14	48	60	0

V-3- THERAPEUTIC FACTORS

V-3-1- SURGERY (Table VII)

Thirteen of the 14 patients had undergone macroscopically complete surgical excision, i.e. enlarged ureteronephrectomy. The mean time to recurrence was 14 months.One of 14 patients with a left nephroblastoma in a bilateral renal nephroblastomatous lesion had undergone partial excision of the left kidney, removing the entire tumour. In this case, the time to recurrence was 48 months.

V-3-2- EXERCISE DIFFICULTIES (Table VII)

Surgical excision was difficult in 7 patients and easy in the other 7.It was noted that the average time to recurrence was shorter, 14 months, for patients with difficult resection, and longer, 26 months, for those with easy resection. The analytical study showed a significant correlation between the time to local recurrence and the difficulty of surgical excision (P=0.0067).

V-3-3- GANGLIONARY COLLECTION (Table VII)

Node sampling was carried out in all patients except 2, who did not have gross adenopathy during surgical exploration. The average time to recurrence was short (9.5 months) in the absence of lymph node sampling, and longer (25.5 months) in the case of lymph node sampling.

Table VII: Time to recurrence and surgical factors.

Observation no.	Recidivism delay (months)	Surgical resection	Difficulty of resection	Node sampling
1	5	complete	Difficult	Yes
2	3	complete	Difficult	Yes
3	8	complete	Difficult	Yes
4	4	complete	Easy	Yes
5	7	complete	Easy	No
6	5	complete	Easy	Yes
7	3	complete	Difficult	Yes
8	11	complete	Easy	Yes
9	4	complete	Difficult	Yes
10	12	complete	Easy	No
11	8	complete	Difficult	Yes
12	12	complete	Easy	Yes
13	25	complete	Difficult	Yes
14	48	partial	Easy	Yes

V-3-4- PRE-OPERATIVE CHEMICAL THERAPY (Table VIII)

All our patients had received pre-operative chemotherapy except one, in whom mesoblastic nephroma was strongly suspected.In 11 patients, partial regression of the renal tumour was 65% on average. One patient showed stability of the lesion and the other an increase in tumour size. In the latter 2 patients, the time to recurrence was 3 months (the shortest time to recurrence in our series). The average time to recurrence was 26 months for patients with partial regression.

V-3-5- POST-OPERATIVE CHEMICAL THERAPY (Table VIII)

All our patients had received postoperative chemotherapy except one, for whom clinical and radiological monitoring was decided. Twelve of the 13 cases had a favourable outcome. One had a local worsening (recurrence of the mass on the follow-up abdominal scan). The time to recurrence was 3 months for patients with local worsening, and 25.5 months on average for patients with a favourable outcome.

Table I: Recurrence factors and response to chemotherapy.

Observation no.	Recidivism delay (months)	Response to pre operating	Response to post-treatment chemotherapy operating
1	5	Regression	Favourable
2	3	Increase	Favourable
3	8	Regression	Favourable
4	4	Regression	Favourable
5	7	-----	-----
6	5	Regression	Favourable
7	3	Stability	Recurrence
8	11	Regression	Favourable
9	4	Regression	Favourable
10	12	Regression	Favourable
11	8	Regression	Favourable
12	12	Regression	Favourable
13	25	Regression	Favourable
14	48	Regression	Favourable

It was noted that the earliest time to recurrence (between 3 and 5 months) was associated in most cases with difficulty in surgical resection.

This delay was also earlier, by 3 months, for patients who were resistant to preoperative chemotherapy (stable or increasing tumour size).

V-4- ANATOMO-PATHOLOGICAL FACTORS (Table IX)

V-4-1- STAGES OF TUMOUR EXTENSION

Six patients had stage I tumour extension, and 8 patients were classified as stage II, III or IV. The average time to recurrence for stage I was 6.7 months, for stage II 26 months, for stage III 6 months and for stage IV 8.3 months. The analytical study showed a significant correlation between the time to local recurrence and the stage of tumour extension (P=0.036). We noted that stage I (in 6 patients) was associated with a fairly short recurrence time (mean recurrence time of 6.7 months). This can be explained by :

-The combination of a blastaematous component and anaplasia in 4 out of 6 cases.

-Difficulties in surgical removal in 2 out of 6 cases.

-The absence of lymph node sampling in 2 cases out of 6.

-Resistance to chemotherapy (stability or worsening of the lesion) in 2 out of 6 cases.

-The absence of pre- or post-operative chemotherapy in one case out of 6 (suspected Bollande tumour).

-Initial tumour size greater than 110 mm in 2 out of 6 cases

V-4-2- HISTOLOGICAL TYPE

The mixed type was the dominant histological type in our series(9patients). Blastematous type was noted in the remaining 5 patients.
The average time to recurrence was shorter for blastematous histological types (7.5 months), and longer for mixed tumours (26 months).
The analytical study did not show a significant correlation between the time to local recurrence and the histological type of tumour (P=0.2433).

V-4-3- UNFAVOURABLE HISTOLOGICAL SIGNS (ANAPLASIA)
Three of the 14 patients had unfavourable histological signs.

The average time to recurrence was very short in the case of anaplasia (3.5 months), and longer in the absence of anaplasia (26.5 months).
The analytical study did not show a significant correlation between time to local recurrence and anaplasia (P=0.231). The earliest time to recurrence (3 or 4 months) was associated with a blastaematous component and anaplasia.

V-4-4- TUMOUR WEIGHT

The tumour weight averaged 1670 grams in the 3 cases where it was mentioned in the pathology report. The time to recurrence was a short 3 months for the 2 patients with tumours weighing 550 grams or more, and longer, 11 months for the patient with a tumour weighing less than 550 grams.

Table IX: Time to recurrence and anatomopathological factors.

Observation no.	Time limit repeat offence (months)	Extension stage	Histological type	Anaplasia	Tumour weight(g)
1	5	IV	Mixed	-	----
2	3	I	Blastematous	+	2800
3	8	IV	Mixed	-	----
4	4	I	Mixed	-	----
5	7	I	Blastematous	-	----
6	5	II	Mixed	-	----
7	3	I	Blastematous	+	1200
8	11	I	Mixed	-	540
9	4	III	Blastematous	+	----
10	12	I	Blastematous	-	----
11	8	III	Mixed	-	----
12	12	IV	Mixed	-	----
13	25	II	Mixed	-	----
14	48	II	Mixed	-	----

DISCUSSION

I- INTRODUCTION

Nephroblastoma or Wilms' tumour is a malignant tumour of the kidney. It reproduces embryonic tissue derived from the metanephros [1, 2, 3, 4]. Nephroblastoma accounts for 5-10% of childhood malignancies. It is the most common abdominal tumour in early childhood, with an average age of 3 to 4 years [1, 2, 5].Certain congenital malformations are associated with an increased risk of nephroblastoma: aniridia, body hemi hypertrophy and genitourinary anomalies (horseshoe kidney, duplicity) [2, 5, 6].

However, most nephroblastomas occur "de novo" in children with no previous history [7].

The development of this tumour is determined by abnormalities (within the tumour cells) in a family of tumour suppressor genes carried by chromosome 11. This gene controls differentiation of the kidney at the embryonic stage [8, 9].

Nephroblastoma is a diagnostic and therapeutic emergency [10], as it progresses very rapidly and can sometimes form a tumour weighing more than 1000 grams.

The diagnosis is made on imaging: ultrasound and abdomino-pelvic CT scan with uroscanner if necessary. This simple radiological work-up is usually sufficient to make the diagnosis of nephroblastoma. It allows treatment to be started without histological evidence, and must be confirmed at a later stage by pathological examination of the excision specimen [3, 6, 7, 11].

Ultrasound or abdomino-pelvic CT scan is essential for accurate assessment of progress with chemotherapy [3, 6, 7, 8, 10, 11].

Treatment is multidisciplinary, combining chemotherapy, surgery and radiotherapy to varying degrees [12, 13, 14]. The prognosis is currently very good, with a cure rate of around 90% [15, 16, 17].Metastasis or local recurrence mainly occurs in the first 2 years after diagnosis, especially for stages III and IV and unfavourable histologies. They should be detected by quarterly surveillance including a clinical examination, chest X-ray and abdominal ultrasound [2, 6, 16, 18, 19]. The prognosis for recurrence remains poor, with a low survival rate [6, 19]. With the aim of improving survival, a number of factors predictive of recurrence have been studied, including clinical, radiological, therapeutic and pathological factors. These factors also make it possible to define groups of patients at high risk of recurrence, to provide them with the most appropriate treatment, to monitor them strictly and to detect any local recurrence at an early stage, thereby ensuring early management [2, 16, 19].

II- INITIAL TUMOUR

II-1- EPIDEMIOLOGY

Nephroblastoma or Wilms' tumour is the most common malignant tumour of the kidney in children (more than 90% of renal tumours in children) [1, 2, 3, 4, 5]. Age at diagnosis varies between 1 and 5 years, with an average of 37 and 43 months for males and females respectively [20, 21, 22]. However, cases of nephroblastoma occurring in adults have been reported [23, 24].The tumour affects both sexes with the same frequency, the sex ratio being close to 1 in different series [6, 5, 8, 14]. A study carried out by Inci Y [15] on 106 patients showed a predominance of males in 58% of cases.

II-2- CLINICAL

Nephroblastoma is most frequently discovered by palpation of an abdominal mass, in 95% of cases [3, 5, 9, 15, 17, 25, 26].This mass is most often discovered by the parents or during a routine medical examination. It may resemble a large spleen or liver. It is often painless, firm, anteriorly developed and rapidly progressive. Clinical examination must be carried out with care, as the tumour is fragile and may rupture [25, 26, 27, 28, 29, 30]. Abdominal pain, haematuria, arterial hypertension and acute abdominal crises due to a traumatic rupture in the peritoneal cavity are also circumstances in which the tumour may be discovered [16, 27, 30, 31]. A study carried out by Mir-Mahmood S. [5] on 55 patients showed that the left side was most often affected (54.5% of cases). Inci Y [15] found the same result, with left-sided involvement in 53% of cases. However, similar right and left renal damage has been observed in several other studies [17, 19, 20, 31].In several studies, nephroblastoma is usually large (mean 110 mm) and sometimes bulky [1, 3, 8, 10, 19, 22, 28].

II-3- RADIOLOGICAL EXAMINATIONS

Medical imaging can be used to make the diagnosis and carry out a full extension assessment, enabling the appropriate therapeutic indications to be chosen [32, 33, 34].It specifies the size of the tumour, its nature, its location, local extension, vascular and lymph node invasion and the search for distant metastases [23, 30, 35]. The PSA shows the existence of a mass syndrome in the form of an opacity projecting onto the renal area and blocking the digestive tract. Calcifications can sometimes be seen (10-15% of cases). The presence of bone lysis suggests a diagnosis of neuroblastoma [3, 6, 12, 33, 34].

Abdominal ultrasound is used to determine the nature, size, location and relationship of the mass. It confirms the retroperitoneal, intrarenal location of the tumour and the echogenic, heterogeneous appearance with patches of necrosis, which is highly suggestive of nephroblastoma [30, 32, 34, 35].

The abdomino-pelvic CT scan confirms the information provided by the ultrasound scan. It clearly shows the renal origin of the tumour and its local or distant extension. It also provides a good study in the case of bilateral tumours. Injection of contrast product enables the vascular time to be studied in search of tumour thrombosis. Urographic images, taken at the same time as the CT scan with injection, show the characteristic opacification of the urinary tract seen in nephroblastoma, with disruption of the normal architecture of the pyelocalic cavities, which appear stretched, deformed or amputated [34, 35].

Abdominal Doppler ultrasound can be used to study the vascularisation of the kidney in search of venous thrombosis [4, 7, 10, 30, 38]. The role of biopsy and its technical procedures are not clearly established in the context of childhood kidney tumours, and there are differences between Anglo-Saxon and American protocols. This is not only the case in European countries, but also within the same protocol, depending in particular on the age of the child. A biopsy may be considered by SIOP teams when the clinical or imaging findings are not consistent with the diagnosis of nephroblastoma: unusual age (over 6 years), notion of infection, presence of calcifications, large adenopathies or lesions, particularly extra-renal. The technical requirements for percutaneous puncture biopsy must be scrupulously respected. Open" surgical biopsy has no a priori indication. On the other hand, any decision to perform a biopsy should only be taken after multidisciplinary consultation, which is particularly necessary in the case of an atypical tumour [36, 37, 38, 39].

II-4- ASSESSMENT OF EXTENSION

The extension work-up includes a search for pulmonary metastases (present from the outset in 20% of cases), which may be visible on a chest X-ray (front and side) or a chest CT scan [30, 39]. Ultrasound and abdominal CT scans can be used to identify hepatic or locoregional metastases and to study the contralateral kidney. Bone metastases are very rare in nephroblastoma (0.8% of cases) and should only be investigated, using bone scintigraphy, if there are suggestive clinical signs [30, 39].

II-5- TREATMENT

Therapeutic advances in nephroblastoma have only been possible thanks to the results of major international multicentre trials conducted mainly by the SIOP in Europe and the NWTS in the United States [40]. The therapeutic strategy of the SIOP protocol depends on the child's age, the stage of extension and the histological type of tumour. After the age of 6 months, children receive pre-operative chemotherapy, with the aim of achieving tumour reduction, reducing the risk of intraoperative tumour rupture and surgical complications. This pre-operative chemotherapy combines Vincristine and Actinomycin D in localised forms, with the addition of Epirubicin in metastatic forms. Children under the age of 6 months are operated on immediately because of the high incidence of mesoblastic nephromas, tumours curable by surgery alone, and the poor tolerance of chemotherapy in this age group. age. Post-operative treatment varies in length and intensity depending on the histological variety and stage of extension of the tumour [5,15, 40, 41, 42].

In the NWTS studies, surgical resection of the primary tumour was the initial treatment for most children. Pre-operative chemotherapy was recommended in certain circumstances, including Wilms' tumour in a single kidney, horseshoe kidney or bilateral tumour, as well as the presence of thrombosis of the IVC or advanced pulmonary metastasis. NWTS uses almost the same chemotherapy combinations as SIOP. Post-operative treatment also depends on the histological type and stage of extension of the tumour [40,43, 44, 45,46].

II-5-1- CHEMOTHERAPY

Chemotherapy has been responsible for spectacular progress in the treatment of nephroblastoma, which is a highly chemosensitive tumour. This is why chemotherapy is used as the first-line treatment strategy for PCOS, in order to reduce tumour volume (tumour reduction of up to 50% of the initial tumour volume), reduce the risk of intraoperative rupture and prevent and treat metastases. This chemotherapy is started on clinical and radiological grounds, without histological evidence [40, 42, 43, 45, 46]. The active drugs are essentially Actinomycin, Adriamycin (Doxorubicin), Vincristine and Oncovin [40, 42, 43, 45]. On the whole, the toxicities of these drugs are tolerable (nausea, vomiting and neutropenia, which are often brief), allowing outpatient treatment to be carried out most of the time [2, 5, 40, 47].

Over the years, SIOP studies have deduced the following:

• SIOP 1: The addition of 6 courses of Actinomycin alone did not improve survival.

• SIOP 2: Post-operative chemotherapy could be reduced from 15 to 6 months.

• SIOP 6: The addition of Doxorubicin improved recurrence-free survival in stages II N+ and III.

• SIOP 9: The addition of a further 4 weeks of preoperative chemotherapy combining Vincristine and Actinomycin did not increase the percentage of stage I disease.

These various studies have shown the prognostic role of histology and have enabled three different groups to be distinguished: a low-risk histology group, an intermediate-risk group and a high-risk group (unfavourable histology). The prognostic role of lymph node involvement has also been studied. This has led to stage II N+ patients being treated in the same way as patients with stage III tumours [1, 7, 40, 47]. Preoperative chemotherapy consists of 4 weekly injections of Vincristine (1.5 mg/m²/cure) and 2 courses of Actinomycin (1.5 mg/m²/cure) spaced 15 days apart (weeks 1 and 3). This is followed 1 week later by surgical excision [1, 40]. The duration of post-operative chemotherapy will depend on the extent of the tumour (surgical staging) and its histological appearance.So for low-risk histologies: no treatment is planned for stage I, whereas for other stages, treatment is identical to that for intermediate histological risk. For intermediate-risk histologies: combination of 2 drugs (Vincristine and Actinomycin) for stage I and 3 drugs (Vincristine, Actinomycin and Epirubicin) for advanced stages, with a duration varying between 18 and 27 weeks.For unfavourable histologies (anaplastic forms) treatment is intensified with the addition of courses combining Ifosfamide-Epirubicin and Carboplatin-Etoposide for 24 weeks [1, 7, 40, 47].

II-5-2- RADIOTHERAPY

Nephroblastoma is one of the most radiosensitive malignant tumours, but the after-effects of irradiation have led to its use being limited to advanced stages. Current indications have been established thanks to various multicentre therapeutic trials [49, 50]. Initially, in the first SIOP trial, radiotherapy was used preoperatively to reduce the risk of intraoperative rupture. This strategy considerably reduced the risk of rupture and increased the number of localised stages. However, due to the significant after-effects of radiotherapy, with a dose of 30 grays, this strategy was superseded by pre-operative chemotherapy. At present, radiotherapy is only given to stage II N+ and III patients with favourable histology, and to stage II N- patients with unfavourable histology. Lung irradiation is performed in the event of incomplete remission of metastases following postoperative chemotherapy [1, 2, 5, 48, 49, 50, 51].

II-5-3- SURGERY

Treatment of nephroblastoma always includes at least one surgical stage [1, 20, 33, 55]. Even as part of a multidisciplinary team, the surgeon's role is not limited to performing the excision procedure specified in the protocol in the best possible way. He shares responsibility with the pathologist for determining the stage of the tumour, which determines post-operative treatment [1, 3, 52, 53, 54]. Nephrorectomy for nephroblastoma remains a major operation involving contact with the large abdominal vessels, with a potential risk of sudden haemorrhage [1, 3, 52, 53, 54]. The reference technique for unilateral forms is an enlarged total ureteronephrectomy [52, 53]. This is an open operation with a wide transperitoneal approach. A transverse supra umbilical incision allows careful exploration and examination of the peritoneal cavity and contralateral kidney, if this has not been well examined by radiological investigations [52, 53, 54, 55]. The renal artery and vein are first ligated, followed by ligation of the ureter flush with the bladder. The hilar lymph nodes and all suspicious regional lymph nodes were removed, without any real lymph node curage. The adrenal gland is removed in the case of superior polar tumours and in the event of invasion of the adrenal gland [56, 57]. The operative specimen, correctly oriented, must be handed over to the pathologist in its entirety, never in pieces. A diagram and/or marker wires are used to indicate areas suspected of being invasive, of crossing the capsule or of adhering to neighbouring organs. The location of lymph nodes taken separately is also indicated on this diagram, as are any suspicious areas [1, 56, 57]. In the case of bilateral tumours or tumours on a single kidney: whether it is a synchronous bilateral tumour, a metachronous contralateral tumour or a tumour on a congenitally single kidney, the strategy is to be as conservative as possible while respecting the imperatives of carcinological safety and urological safety. Preoperative chemotherapy is continued until maximum tumour shrinkage has been achieved. Polar tumours or small tumours may benefit, depending on their location, from a regulated partial nephrectomy involving a "slice" of kidney, a wedge-shaped resection involving a small amount of healthy parenchyma around the tumour and, in extreme cases, a lumpectomy flush with the kidney. the tumour pseudocapsule. In these cases of partial resection, an extemporaneous microscopic examination of the margins is necessary. In this case, a very massive tumour and/or one invading the entire hilum or sinus of the kidney requires total nephrectomy [55].

II-5-4- ANATOMOPATHOLOGY

This embryonic malignant tumour develops from the nephrogenic blastema. The tumour cells have several differentiation pathways, reproducing the histology of the developing kidney. The tumour is grey, pink or yellowish, and is surrounded by a pseudocapsule. It is soft or firm in consistency, depending on the amount of stromal contingent, and may be cystic, haemorrhagic or necrotic. There are 3 contingents in the usual form: blastaematous, epithelial and stromal [1, 20, 25, 48]. The blastémate contingent consists of sheets of undifferentiated cells with round or oval nuclei containing a small nucleolus. Nuclear superimposition and mitosis are frequent. The architecture is diffuse, nodular or "serpentine". The mixed type is the association of the 3 contingents in close percentages [1, 20, 25, 48].Anaplasia may be present in each of the 3 contingents and is defined by the presence of polypoid multipolar mitoses, hyperchromatism and a 3-fold increase in nuclear size. Anaplasia may be focal or diffuse (1, 25, 48).

II-6- PROGNOSIS

The management strategy for renal tumours has evolved in divergent ways (from 1970 to the present day) under the influence of the NWTS group and the SIOP. In recent years, these 2 groups have come closer together, both through the use of similar histological classifications and through the satisfactory results obtained [17]. With advances in treatment, the prognosis for the disease is currently very good, with a cure rate of around 90% [2, 5, 7, 9, 10, 15, 20]. In other studies, the survival rate varies between 72.4% and 98.5% of cases [30, 33, 45, 50, 53].

II-7- SURVEILLANCE

Monitoring usually involves a full clinical examination, chest X-ray and abdominal ultrasound. The closer the patient is to the end of treatment, the more frequent the monitoring. is recent (every 2 to 3 months for the first 2 or 3 years). However, the precise details of this monitoring are still under discussion [1, 7, 34, 50].

III- TUMOUR RECURRENCE

Local recurrence is defined as recurrence of the mass in the original tumour bed, retroperitoneally or within the abdominal cavity [52].

III-1- CIRCUMSTANCES OF DISCOVERY

In several studies, recurrence was discovered at quarterly follow-up radiological examinations in 82 to 97% of cases [1, 2, 5, 6, 52, 55, 58]. In our series, radiological surveillance was the reason for the discovery of recurrence in 86% of cases.

III-2- TIME BETWEEN DETERMINATION OF RECURRENCE AND NEPHRECTOMY

The study by Inci Y [15] showed an average delay of 39 months. Whereas the study by Eun S. [5] and Mir-Mahmood S. [16] found a shorter mean time to recurrence of 11 and 13 months respectively. In 2012, a Korean study by So-Young L. [7] noted that most tumour recurrences (86% of cases) occur within the first 2 years after diagnosis of the disease. In contrast, late recurrences, defined as 5 years after the initial diagnosis, are extremely rare events.In the same study, the author reported the longest time to local tumour recurrence, 25 years, in one case. To explain this long delay in recurrence, So-Young L. referred to a study by Senetta [7], who found that preoperative chemotherapy of the initial tumour stimulates tumour differentiation, leading to tumour maturation and removal of immature tumour components. Immature tumour components are more sensitive to pre-operative chemotherapy. Eradication of the high-quality immature component and induction of a high degree of differentiation therefore prolongs the time to recurrence. In our series, the mean time to recurrence was 25.5 months.

III-3- LOCATION OF RECURRENT TUMOURS

Most tumour recurrences occur in the lung, with local recurrences being rarer [2, 5, 7, 52].Isolated pulmonary recurrences are the most frequent sites of recurrence. They accounted for 41% in a study carried out by Inci Y [15]. They are followed by liver, lymph node and bone metastases. In a study carried out by Robert C. [52] on 2482 patients, the frequency of local recurrence was 4%.The frequency of local recurrence associated with a metastasis varied between 15 and 20% in several studies, including 50% of pulmonary metastases [9, 16, 38, 52]. In our study, the incidence of local recurrence was 12%. The incidence of metastases was 36%, 80% of which were pulmonary.

III-4- TREATMENT OF TUMOUR RECURRENCE

III-4-1- CHEMOTHERAPY

Given that local recurrences are rare, no study has established a clear consensus on the treatment of recurrences [38]. A study carried out by Robert C. [52] on 2482 cases concluded that patients who had received more drugs (in number and dose) during chemotherapy treatment of the initial tumour had a poor prognosis for recurrence. Also, those who had received Doxorubicin (Adriamycin) during the initial treatment had a lower incidence of relapse than those who did not, but this difference was not statistically significant. In our series, 23% of patients had received Adriamycin (Doxorubicin) in combination with Vincristine and Actinomycin during preoperative chemotherapy of the initial tumour. The mean time to recurrence was short at 5.5 months, whereas it was longer at 26 months for patients who had not received Adriamycin. Another study by Eun S. [16], on 98 patients, showed an improvement in the prognosis of tumour recurrence with the introduction of new therapies: ifosfamide, etoposide and carboplatin. The latter had demonstrated their efficacy, with a response rate in monotherapy varying between 42 and 53%, and a response rate in combination of (Ifosfamide and Etoposide or Etoposide and Carboplatin) between 55 and 83%. However, none of these approaches improved long-term survival by more than 30% [16, 58, 59, 60].In 2009, Filippo S. [38] concluded that high-dose therapy had a role in the treatment of recurrence, with an overall survival rate of up to 60-73%. In this study, prognostic indicators (histology and tumour stage) were adopted as inclusion criteria for the application of high-dose therapy to patients at high risk of non-response to conventional-dose chemotherapy. According to Filippo S. [38], there was an improvement in results compared with published historical data, even though there was no consensus regarding the contribution of high-dose chemotherapy. All in all, analysis of recent paediatric studies looking at the use of chemotherapy with a variety of treatment protocols shows that it is undeniably beneficial. The aim for the future is to try to avoid recurrences by identifying at-risk groups and helping them with more appropriate treatments and strict monitoring after remission [16, 19, 38, 52, 61, 62, 63, 64]. In our study, 93% of our patients had received pre-operative chemotherapy, of whom 77% had achieved an average partial regression of the tumour of 65%.

III-4-2- SURGERY

Recurrence surgery using the old approach is always indicated if the mass occupying the renal cavity is resectable, and if the patient's clinical condition allows it [60, 64, 65, 66]. Surgical excision must be as complete as possible [60, 63, 67, 68]. In our series, 78% of patients were operable (resectable tumour), and gross resection was complete in all patients.

III-4-3- ANATOMOPATHOLOGICAL EXAMINATION

In 2007, a study by Senetta [7] divided tumour recurrences into 2 groups according to their histological differentiation: a group of immature, undifferentiated tumours and another group of mature, highly differentiated tumours. According to this study, the division was due to whether or not preoperative chemotherapy was taken during treatment of the initial tumour. Patients who had received pre-operative chemotherapy no longer had immature elements in their tumours. These patients had a longer time to recurrence. In our study, among 93% of our patients who had received pre-operative chemotherapy, 28.5% of cases had a change in histological type, from mixed type to chemotherapy. predominantly blastematous. The average time to recurrence was relatively short, at 8.5 months. Patients who did not initially present with anaplasia retained the same histological characteristics.

III-5- PROGNOSIS

Several studies had noted that the survival rate of children after recurrence was low, varying between 35 and 50% of cases [68, 69, 70, 71].In the 1998 study by Robert C. [52] of 2482 patients, 4% of cases had relapsed, with a survival rate (2 years after relapse) of 43%. In 2006, the study by Eun S. [16], on 98 patients, 12% of cases had recurred with a survival rate of 40.9%. The prognosis for a recurrent Wilms' tumour is generally better if the tumour has the following characteristics: favourable histology, stage I at diagnosis, has not had Doxorubicin-based chemotherapy or radiotherapy, and recurs at least 12 months after initial diagnosis [54].In our series, of the 14 cases studied, 72% had a favourable outcome with complete disappearance of the recurrent local tumour and metastases. The mean follow-up time for the 14 patients was 47.5 months. However, 28% of cases had an unfavourable outcome.

IV- FACTORS PREDICTIVE OF RECIDIVISM

IV-1- CLINICAL FACTORS

IV-1-1- AGE

Being very young is a more favourable prognostic factor. Children aged less than 24 months have a better prognosis than older children [54].

A study by Inci Y [15] and another by Robert C [52] concluded that patient age at diagnosis was a prognostic factor when considered alone, with an increased risk of local recurrence in older children (aged 4 years). In these 2 studies, the effect of age failed to achieve a statistically significant correlation. In other studies, such as that by Mir-Mahmood S. [5], and that by Eun S. [16], the age of patients was not considered to be a predictive factor for recurrence. In our series, more than half the patients (57%) were under or equal to 3 years of age. Thus, patients older than 3 years had earlier recurrences than those younger than or equal to 3 years. We also noted that the oldest patient (9 years) in our study had the earliest recurrence time (3 months).

IV-1-2- SEX

The patient's sex has never been considered to be a predictive factor for local recurrence, and this has been the case in various studies [2, 52, 72].

In the 2 analytical studies carried out by Mir-Mahmood S. [5] and Inci Y. [15], there was no significant correlation between the time to recurrence and the sex of the patients. In our series, male patients recurred earlier than female patients, with no statistically significant correlation.

IV-2- RADIOLOGICAL FACTORS

IV-2-1- SIZE OF THE INITIAL TUMOUR

Small tumours are associated with a more favourable prognosis than large tumours [54]. The study by Inci Y. [15] and another by Eun S. [16] concluded that the incidence of recurrence was related to the initial tumour size. Eun S. [16] found that tumours larger than 110 mm recurred earlier than those smaller than 110 mm. In 2012, a Korean study by So-young L. [7] showed a statistically significant correlation between the time to recurrence and the size of the initial tumour ($P = 0.0034$). In our series, we came to the same conclusion.

IV-2-2- DISTANT METASTASES

Several studies agreed that the initial presence of a distant metastasis was a significant predictor of recurrence [5, 15, 52]. In the study carried out by Inci Y [5] on 106 patients, 58% of cases with initial distant metastases had recurred. Also, in a study by Robert C. [52] of 2482 patients, 52% of recurrent patients had distant metastases from the outset. In our study, 21% of patients had metastatic disease. The average time to recurrence was considered to be fairly early (8.5 months).

IV-3- THERAPEUTIC FACTORS

IV-3-1- SURGICAL RESECTION

A study by Robert C. [52] and one by Andrew M. [6] showed that the presence of macroscopic residues in the surgical resection margin was a predictive factor for local recurrence. In our study, an extended ureteronephrectomy was performed in all but one patient. The resection was considered macroscopically complete in all patients. The mean time to recurrence for the 14 patients was a relatively long 25.5 months.

IV-3-2- OPERATING DIFFICULTIES

The study carried out by Robert C. [52] showed that abdominal recurrence was closely linked to the difficulty of surgical excision. The analytical study showed a significant correlation between the time to recurrence and the difficulty of surgical excision. In our study, surgical resection was difficult in 7 patients (50%), but there was no invasion of the renal capsule. The time to recurrence was earlier in patients whose surgical resection was difficult.

IV-3-3- TUMOUR RUPTURE

In a study by Eun S. [16], surgical rupture was always associated with local recurrence. The time to recurrence was fairly early. In 2009, Filippo S. [38] concluded that surgical rupture of the tumour should be avoided by the surgeon, as patients who had an intraoperative capsular break had an earlier recurrence time than those who did not.

IV-3-4- LYMPH NODE SAMPLING

Extensive lymph node dissection of Wilms' tumour has not been recommended, although lymph node sampling was strongly indicated in the study by Weirich A. [40]. The study carried out by Ali T. [30] on 42 cases concluded that lymph node dissection did not seem to influence survival or the rate of local recurrence. However, the absence of lymph node sampling may lead to an underestimation of the stage of tumour extension, resulting in inadequate treatment of the child and frequent local recurrence. In our study, lymph node sampling was performed in all but 2 patients (because no suspicious adenopathies were evident on surgical exploration). The time to recurrence was relatively early in the absence of lymph node sampling (9.5 months).

IV-3-5- PRE-OPERATIVE CHEMOTHERAPY

Proponents of preoperative chemotherapy (SIOP) suggest that it helps to reduce tumour volume and the risk of intraoperative rupture, as well as preventing the occurrence of metastases. Thus, preoperative chemotherapy helps to reduce mortality and morbidity [73, 74].Robert C. [52] and Mir-Mahmoud S. [5] concluded that pre-operative chemotherapy greatly facilitated surgery (considerable regression of the initial tumour volume). In 2007, Senetta [7] defined 2 groups, one having received preoperative chemotherapy and the other not. She concluded that initial chemotherapy contributes to the maturation and differentiation of the initial tumour, which prolongs the time to recurrence. In our series, after chemotherapy, partial regression averaged 65% in 76% of cases, with a fairly long average time to recurrence of 26 months. This delay was much earlier (3 months) in patients who had not responded to chemotherapy (stability or worsening of the lesion).

IV-3-6- POST-OPERATIVE CHEMOTHERAPY

Several studies have concluded that postoperative chemotherapy helps to increase relapse-free survival [52, 53, 55, 73].Jonathan C [58], in a study of 81 patients, and Silvio T [59], in a study of 53 patients, agreed on the need for postoperative chemotherapy, with the duration and combination of drugs depending on the prognostic criteria (stage and histology). In our series, 71.4% of patients had a favourable outcome after chemotherapy, with an average time to recurrence of 25.5 months. One patient out of 14 had a local worsening and thus had the earliest recurrence time (3 months).

IV-4- ANATOMO-PATHOLOGICAL FACTORS

IV-4-1- STAGES OF TUMOUR EXTENSION

The earlier the stage, the better the prognosis. A Wilms' tumour that has spread to lymph nodes or other sites has a poorer prognosis [54]. A study by Almamy Cisse B. [2], another by Mir-Mahmood S. [5], and other studies [6, 52, 75, 76] agreed that the stage of tumour extension is the most important prognostic factor. Since the appropriate therapy and prognosis depend on the stage of the tumour, accurate patient classification is imperative and includes histological evaluation of the regional lymph nodes [77]. The study by Robert C. [52] and that by Eun S. [16] noted that local recurrence was most frequently observed in patients with stage III or IV tumour extension.

In our study, we noted that 6 patients had stage I and 8 patients had stage II, III or IV. Stages III and IV had a relatively early mean time to recurrence (6 months and 8.3 months respectively). However, stage II had a longer recurrence time of 26.5 months. Paradoxically, stage I was associated with a relatively early mean time to recurrence (6.5 months). This was essentially explained by the association with unfavourable histological factors.

IV-4-2- HISTOLOGICAL TYPE

Nephroblastoma with a predominance of epithelial cells is thought to be less aggressive [75, 76]. All the studies carried out agreed that the blastaematous component is a poor prognostic factor, in particular the study by Robert C. [52] and that by Inci Y. [15]. In the study by Delarue A. [17], the predominantly blastematous histological type was classified as high risk.In our study, the mixed type was the most frequent histological type (64%). Patients with a mixed type had a longer mean time to recurrence (26 months) than those with a predominantly blastematous component (7.5 months).

IV-4-3- UNFAVOURABLE HISTOLOGICAL SIGNS (ANAPLASIA)

Anaplastic nephroblastoma accounts for around 5% of childhood kidney tumours, and increases in frequency with age [9]. Anaplasia is the abnormal loss of certain cell differentiation characteristics, with no return to the primary cell state. It is thought to be a chemotherapy-resistant clone [9]. The grade of Wilms' tumour is a very important predictor of recurrence. Tumours with favourable histology (absence of anaplasia) have a better prognosis than those with unfavourable histology (presence of anaplasia). Anaplasia is associated with higher recurrence rates and a poorer prognosis [54]. The prognosis for anaplastic tumours is particularly poor [52, 75, 77].

In the study by Delarue A [17], patients with anaplastic tumours were classified as being at high risk of recurrence.In our series, 21.4% of our patients had unfavourable histological signs, with a mean time to early recurrence of 3.5 months.

IV-4-4- TUMOUR WEIGHT

In the study by Robert C. [52], tumour weight was a significant prognostic factor associated with abdominal recurrence. Tumours weighing less than 550 grams were considered to be at low risk of recurrence. In our series, tumours weighing more than 550 grams had an early recurrence time of 3 months.

TOTAL

It has recently been recognised that the stage of tumour extension (SIOP) alone is not sufficient to accurately identify all patients at risk of recurrence, and that other factors need to be taken into consideration, such as patient age, tumour weight, and response to chemotherapy [75]. In addition, there are few publications in the literature concerning therapeutic regimens and chemotherapy protocols for the treatment of recurrent nephroblastoma tumours [73, 72, 75].

CONCLUSION

Nephroblastoma or Wilms' tumour is the most common malignant renal tumour in children aged between 1 and 5 years. Its prognosis has been significantly improved thanks to therapeutic advances, with a cure rate of up to 90%. Local recurrence may occur within 2 years of diagnosis. Local recurrence is defined as recurrence of the mass in the original tumour bed, retroperitoneally or within the abdominal cavity. It poses the problem of its aetiology, which is multi-factorial, represented essentially by: under-classification of the tumour, inadequate pre- or post-operative chemotherapy, surgical error (tumour rupture, failure to resect peritoneal-diaphragmatic or parietal residues), and unfavourable histology. The survival rate after recurrence is also low, varying between 35 and 50%. All the authors agree on the usefulness of studying the recurrence factors that need to be taken into consideration in order to be able to accurately identify all patients at high risk of recurrence. The aim is to improve the cure rate in groups at risk of recurrence and help them with more appropriate treatments. Our hope is that this work will be a prelude to in-depth multicentre research into new active chemotherapeutic agents and new, more appropriate treatment regimens to improve the prognosis and survival rate of recurrent patients.

APPENDIX

Stages of tumour extension adopted according to SIOP 2001.

Stage I: Localised tumour not extending beyond the renal capsule and not invading the fat of the renal hilum.

Stage II: Localised tumour, extending beyond the limits of the kidney (peri-renal fat, thrombosis of the renal vein, involvement of the renal hilum, etc.), or biopsied tumour with macroscopically total resection.

Stage III: Tumour disseminated in the abdomen by a non-haematogenous route (peritoneal implants, lymph node invasion of peri-aortic chains, invasion of neighbouring organs or tumour ruptured in the abdomen) with residual tumour after nephrectomy.

Stage IV: Tumours with haematogenous metastases.

Stage V: Bilateral tumours.

BIBLIOGRAPHY

1. Chastagner P, Fournet J, Doz F, Gauthier F. Kidney tumours in children.
EMC. Paris: Elsevier, Paediatrics, 4-088-D-10; 2013

2. Almamy Cisse B. Study of the epidemiological aspects of Nephroblastoma in the paediatric ward.
Th D Méd, Mali, 2008.

3. B. Brichard. Nephroblastoma.
Webhosttest.uclouvain.be/sites/oncop/rw/page2/page1/assets/nephroblastoma.pdf, accessed 25 January 2013.

4. Pontual L, Lyonnet S, Amiel J. Developmental abnormalities and predisposition to childhood tumours. Arch Pediatr. 2010; 17: 1220-7.

5. Mir-Mahmood S, Ahmad K, Alireza M, Naser S, Omid A. Wilms tumor: A 10 year's retrospective study. Arch Iranian Med. 2007; 10: 65-9.

6. Andrew M. Wilms tumor. Curr Opin Pediatr. 2009; 21: 357-64.

7. So-Young L, Kyu-Rae K, Jung-Yeol P, Jae Y. Wilms tumor with long delayed recurrence: 25 years after initial treatment.
Korean J Urol. 2012; 53: 288-92.

8. Dominique P. Nephroblastoma or Wilms' tumour. www-sante.ujf-grenoble.fr/SANTE/, accessed on 23 January 2013.

9. Lemerle J, Tournade M. Nephroblastoma (Wilms tumor) Rev Prat. 1993; 43: 2192-6.

10. Landolsi A, Ben Fatma L, Kallel K, Gharbi O, Zakhama A, Golli M, et al. Nephroblastoma in central region of Tunisian clinical and histological study and prognostic factors. Ann Urol. 2003; 37: 164-9.

11. Aloui-Kasbi N, Felah S, Bellagha I, Barsaoui S, Hammou A. Imaging of kidney tumors in children.
J Pédiatr Puéricul.2004; 17: 34-40.

12. Nouira F, Sarrai N, Ghorbel S, Med Sghair Y, Khemakhem R, Chariag A et al. Indications for nephrectomy in children: What has changed? Tunis Méd. 2010; 88: 70-5.

13. Habrand JL, Oberlin O, Pein F, Leblanc T, Levy-Piedbois C, Doz F. Chemotherapy combinations in childhood tumours. Cancer Radiother. 1998; 2: 752-9.

14. Lemerle J, Tournade M, Pein F. Nephroblastoma: A model for chemosensitive childhood cancers. Bull. Acad. Natle Méd. 1998; 182: 1231-46.

15. Inci Y, Lebriz Y, Alp Ö, Hilmi A, Tiraje C, Nur D. Multidisciplinary approach to Wilms tumor: 18 years of experience.
Jpn J Clin Oncol. 2000; 30: 17-20.

16. Eun S, Hyoung J, Hee Y, Hyo S. Improved survival in patients with recurrent Wilms tumor: The experience of the Seoul national university children's hospital.
J Korean Med Sci. 2006; 21: 436-40.

17. Delarue A, Coze C, Gorincour G, Bouvier C, Murraciole X. Kidney tumours in children.
EMC. Paris: Elsevier, Pediatrics, 4-088-D-10; 2007.
18. Ekenze S, Agugua-Obianyo N, Odetunde O. The challenge of nephroblastoma in a developing country.
Ann Oncol. 2006; 17: 1598-600.

19. Kathleen A, Veronica V. Towards an understanding of Wilms tumor. Int. J. Exp. Pathol. 1994; 75: 147-55.
20. Illingworth R, Morris J, Pearson D, Barbor P, Beck J, Bloom H et al. Management of nephroblastoma in childhood.
Arch Dis Child. 1978; 53: 112-9.

21. Maura O, Mark K, James R, Gregory H. Progress in childhood cancer: 50 years of research collaboration, a report from the children's oncology group.
Semin Oncol. 2008; 35: 484-93.

22. Catherine P, Christelle D. Childhood cancers with a good prognosis. Rev Prat. 2007; 57: 1070-6.
23. Moutou C, Hochez J, Chompret A, Tournade M, Le Bihan C, Zucker J et al. The French Wilms tumor study: no clear evidence for cancer prone families.J Med Genet. 1994; 31: 429-34.

24. Buzelin F, Heloury Y, Moreau A, Nomballais M, Lenne Y. Nephroblastomatosis and Wilms' tumour, case report.
Arch Anat Cytol Pathol. 1992; 40 (5-6): 324-8.

25. Okoko A, Ekhouya Bowassa G, Oko A, Mbika-Cardorelle A, Moyen G.
Epidemiology of palpable abdominal masses in children in Brazzaville. Arch Pédiatr. 2012 ; 19 :878-9.
26. Coulomb A. Diagnosis of abdominal tumours in children: pathologist's data.

Arch Pediatr. 2012; 19: 222-3.

27. Cecilia A, Susan P, Patricia A, Janice T, Yevgeny G, Norman E. Early and late mortality after diagnosis of wilms tumor.
J Clin Oncol. 2009; 27: 1304-9.

28. Jason A, Andrew J, Erin H, Colin A, Chase T, Janene P et al. Race disparities in Wilms tumor incidence and biology.
J Surg Res. 2011; 170: 112-9.

29. Han J, Kwon S, Won S, Shin Y, Ko J, Lyu C. Comprehensive clinical follow-up of late effects in childhood cancer survivors shows the need for early and well-timed intervention.
Ann Oncol. 2009; 20: 1170-7.

30. Ali T, Mahmoud P, Hamidreza A, Reza B, Nasim Z, Behrang A. Correlation between size of renal cell carcinoma and its grade, stage, and histological subtype.
Urol J. 2007; 4: 10-3.

31. Marilia F, Gulnar A, Silva M. Prognosis for patients with unilateral Wilms tumor in Rio de Janeiro, Brazil, 1990-2000.
Rev Saúde Pública. 2005; 39: 1-7.

32. Thomas M, Robert Y, Kelley W. Best cases from the AFIP, anaplastic Wilms tumor: Radiologic and pathologic findings.
RadioGraphics. 2004; 24: 1709-13.

33. Theodore L. Atypical presentation of Wilms tumor: Evaluation and early diagnosis. J Natl Med Assoc. 1998; 90: 51-3.
34. Hervé J, Anne M, Sue C, Catherine M. Imaging in unilateral Wilms tumor. Pediatr Radiol. 2008; 38: 18-29.

35. Regaya N. Contribution to the study of renal tumours. Retrospective anatomical-clinical and immunohistochemical study of 43 cases. Th D Méd, Tunis; 2004.

36. Harif M, Barsaoui S, Benchekroun S, Boccon-Gibod L, Bouhas R, Doumbé P, et al. Treatment of childhood cancer in Africa: Preliminary results of the French-African Pediatric oncology group.
Arch Pédiatr.2005; 12: 851-3.

37. Lisa H, Bernardo H, Richard M, Sharon M, Joyce E, Oscar M et al. Pediatric renal masses: Wilms tumor and beyond.
RadioGraphics. 2000; 20: 1585-603.

38. **Filippo S, Kathy P, Cristophe B, Jan K, Sandro D, Norbert G**. Value and difficulties of a common European strategy for recurrent Wilms tumor.
Expert Rev. Anticancer Ther. 2009; 9: 693-6.

39. **Peter F, Fernando A, Michael L, James R, Daniel M, Paul E et al.**
Hepatic metastasis at diagnosis in patients with Wilms tumor is not an independent adverse prognostic factor for stage IV Wilms tumor. A report from the children's oncology group/ National Wilms tumor study group.
Ann Surg. 2009; 250: 642-8.

40. **Weirich A, Ludwig R, Graf N, Abel U, Leuschner I, Vujanic G Et al.**
Survival in Nephroblastoma treated according to the trial and study SIOP-9/GPOH with respect to relapse and morbidity.
Ann Oncol. 2004; 15: 808-20.

41. **Jerzy N, Katarzyna T, Wojciech M, Anna S.** Is the SIOP-2001 classification of renal tumors of childhood accurate with regard to prognosis? A problem revisited.
Arch Med Sci. 2012; 4: 684-9.

42. **Karen D, Daniel M, Najat C.** Late effects of treatment for Wilms tumor.
Pediatr Hematol Oncol. 2009; 26: 407-13.

43. **Piotr P, Andrzej K, Adam M, Katarzyna P, Jacek Z.** Potential role of PET-CT in chemotherapy efficacy assessment and recurrence diagnosis in a patient with a Wilms tumor.
Nucl Med Rev. 2011; 14: 33-5.

44. **Bryan L, Jeffrey M, Jeffrey S, Jamie R, Nita L, Anne Z et al.**
Dactinomycin and Vincristine toxicity in the treatment of childhood cancer: A retrospective study from the children's oncology group.
Pediatr Blood Cancer. 2011; 57: 252-7.

45. **Gauthier F.** Recent developments in renal tumour diseases in children: the role of the paediatric surgeon. Prog Urol. 2001 ; 11 : 109-12.

46. **Monikal L, Jeffrey S.** Current therapy for Wilms tumor.Oncologist. 2005; 10: 815-26.

47. **Thorsten S, Bastian G, Hans-Jürgen S.** Effects of chemotherapy on the cytogenetic constitution of Wilms tumor.
Clin Cancer Res. 2005; 11: 4382-7.

48. **Norman E, Bruce J, Gerald M, John A, Michael L, Robert C et al.**
Radiation therapy for favorable histology Wilms tumor: Prevention of flank recurrence did not improve survival on national Wilms tumor studies.

Int J Radiat Oncol Biol Phys. 2006; 65: 203-9.

49. Chambers E. Radiotherapy in pediatric practice. Arch Dis Child. 1991; 66: 1090-92.

50. Baez F, Fossati Bellani F, Ocampo E, Conter V, Flores A, Gutierrez T, Malta A et al. Treatment of childhood Wilms tumor without radiotherapy in Nicaragua.
Ann Oncol. 2002; 13: 944-8.

51. Hisham H, Emmad E, Mohamed M. Wilms tumor: The experience of the pediatric unit of Kasr El-Aini center of radiation oncology and nuclear medicine (NEMROCK).
J Egypt. Nat. Cancer Inst. 2005; 17: 308-14.

52. Robert C, Katherine A, Michael L, Gerald M, Janice T, Giulio J et al. Surgery-related factors and local recurrence of Wilms tumor in national Wilms tumor.
Ann Surg. 1998; 229: 292-7.

53. Ibrahim Daradka. Indications for nephrectomy in children: A report on 119 cases. Saudi J Kidney Dis Transpl. 2012; 23: 1221-6.

54. Dome J, Perlman E. Wilms' tumour: prognosis and survival.

www.cancer.ca/fr-ca/cancer-information/cancer-type/wilms-tumour/prognosis-and- survival/?region=nb, accessed on 9 June 2013.

55. Andrew M, Dana W, Deborah P, Jesse J, Matthew J, Fredric A et al. The feasibility and outcome of nephron-sparing surgery for children with bilateral Wilms tumor: The St. Jude Children's Research hospital experience: 1999-2006. Cancer.2008; 112: 2060-70.

56. Babai S. La néphroblastomatose chez l'enfant à propos de 2 cas. Th D Méd, Monastir; 2001.

57. Mitchell C, Morris J, Kelsey A, Vujanic G, Marsden B, Shannon R et al. The treatment of Wilms tumor: results of the United Kingdom Children's Cancer Study Group (UKCCSG) second Wilms tumor study.
Br J Cancer. 2000; 83: 602-8.

58. Jonathan C, Dionne A, Carlos R, Caleb P. Contemporary use of nephron-sparing surgery for children with malignant renal tumors at freestanding children's hospitals. Urology.2011; 78: 422-6.

59. Jonathan C, Richard A, Thomas J, Christine M, Douglas A, Stephen A et al. B7-H1 Expression in Wilms tumor: Correlation with tumor biology and disease recurrence. J Urol. 2008; 179: 1954-60.

60. **Silvio T, Adauto J, Haylton J, Elvis T, Luis F, Edson L et al.** Results of novel strategies for treatment of Wilms tumor.
Int Braz J Urol. 2007; 33: 195-203.

61. **Maurer K, Heitger A, Schwaighofer H, Fink F, Niederwieser D.** Double high-dose chemotherapy with autologous peripheral stem cell rescue in relapsed Wilms tumor. Bone Marrow Transplant. 1997; 20: 1111-3.

62. **Huda R, Mohamed S, Ashraf H.** Role of CT in assessment of unresectable Wilms tumor response after preoperative chemotherapy in pediatrics.
Thescientificworldjournal. 2008; 8: 661-9.

63. **Kremens B, Gruhn B, Klingebiel T, Hasan C, Laws H, Koscielniak E et al.** High- dose chemotherapy with autologous stem cell rescue in children with nephroblastoma. Bone Marrow Transplant. 2002; 30: 893-8.

64. **Michael L, Kevin C, Norman E, Janice T, Jami M, Craig W et al.** Management and outcome of inoperable Wilms tumor: A report of national Wilms tumor study.
Ann Surg. 1994; 220: 683-90.

65. **Abu-Ghosh A, Krailo M, Goldman S, Slack R, Davenport V, Morris E et al.** Ifosfamide, Carboplatin and Etoposide in children with poor-risk relapsed Wilms tumor: a Children's Cancer Group report.
Ann Oncol. 2002; 13: 460-9.

66. **Norman E, San-San O, Bruce J, Gerald M, John A, Michael L et al.** Doxorubicin for favorable histology, stage II-III Wilms tumor: Results from the national Wilms tumor studies. Cancer. 2004; 101: 1072-80.

67. **Annemieke I, Leo M, Marry M, Anjo J.** Behavioral and educational limitations after chemotherapy for childhood acute lymphoblastic leukemia or Wilms tumor. Cancer. 2006; 106: 2067-75.

68. **Catherine M, Hervé J, Oystein E, Joanna B, Anne M.** Bilateral disease and new trends in Wilms tumor. Pediatr Radiol. 2008; 38: 30-9.

69. **Hervé J, Gudrun S, Sabine S, Sylvie H, Pascale P, Liliane B et al.** Preoperative Wilms tumor rupture: A retrospective study of 57 patients. Cancer. 2008; 113: 202-13.

70. **Chiang-Ching H, Samantha G, Norman B, Colleen C, Simone T, Irene B et al.** Predicting relapse in favorable histology Wilms tumor using gene expression analysis: A report from the renal tumor committee of the children's oncology group. Clin Cancer Res. 2009; 15: 1770-8.

71. **Debra J, Gian G, Julian G, Donald A.** Distinctive properties of an

anaplastic Wilms tumor and its associated epithelial cell line. Am J Pathol. 1994; 144: 1023-34.

72. Dominique B, Julie L, Gudrun S, Isabelle Z, Liliane B, Monique F et al. High Cyclin E staining index in blastemal, stromal or epithelial cells is correlated with tumor aggressiveness in patients with Nephroblastoma. www.plosone.org, accessed on 23 January 2013.

73. Jean-Jacques Voigt. Cotran, Kumar, Collins. Wilms' Tumour. 3ème ed. Italia: Piccin; 2000.

74. Lilian M, Ricardo J, Maria T, Vicente O, Joao G, Miguel S. Intracaval and Intracardiac extension of Wilms tumor. The influence of preoperative chemotherapy on surgical morbidity. Int Braz J Urol. 2007; 33: 683-9.

75. Robert C, James R, Norman E, Elizabeth J, Bruce B, Michael L et al. Long-term outcomes of infants with very low risk Wilms tumor treated with surgery alone on national Wilms tumor study -5. Ann Surg. 2010; 251: 555-8.

76. John A, Daniel M, Gerald H, James R, Jeffrey S, Paul E. Outcomes of children with favorable histology Wilms tumor and peritoneal implants treated on national Wilms tumor studies.Int J Radiat Oncol Biol Phys. 2010; 77: 554-8.

77. Conrad V, James A, Norman E, Jeffrey S, Grundy P, Elizabeth J et al. Anthropomorphic measurements and event free survival in patients with favorable histology Wilms tumor: A report from the Children's Oncology group. Pediatr Blood Cancer. 2009; 52: 254-8.

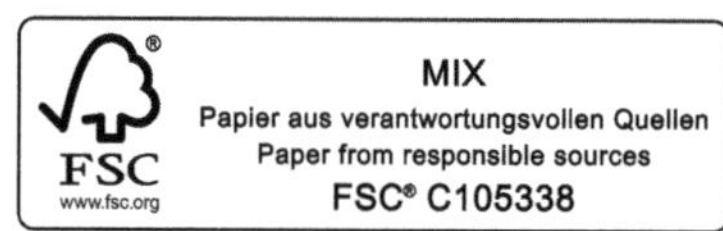

Printed by Books on Demand GmbH, Norderstedt / Germany